Bibliographic information published by the German National Library:

The German National Library lists this publication in the National Bibliography; detailed bibliographic data are available on the Internet at http://dnb.dnb.de .

Imprint:

Print and binding: Books on Demand GmbH, Norderstedt Germany
ISBN: 9783668455269

This book at GRIN:

http://www.grin.com/en/e-book/366636/designing-a-research-compliance-program

Ernestoh Khomu

Designing a Research Compliance Program

GRIN Publishing

Designing a Research Compliance Program

After the management of a healthcare organization tasks the VC of healthcare systems with forming a research compliance department, there are many consideration the executive must make in order to be effective in that capacity. As part of the large organization involved in among other activities healthcare, various ethical issues arise that necessitate the creation of such a department. However, the process is not easy as many considerations have to be made. This paper follows the process of the creation of a Research Compliance Program through an investigation of the process or designing and implementing a Research Compliance Department. The process intends to use a distinct set of considerations that not only form the basic processes of forming the department, but also understanding the operations of the Program. These considerations include who the compliance department answers to, the primary ethical issues involved, how the department intends to maintain oversight, the tools and approaches applicable as well as their applicability, and to assimilate all personnel involved into the notion of additional oversight.

HOW THE RESEARCH COMPLIANCE DEPARTMENT WILL FIT INTO THE ORGANIZATIONAL STRUCTURE

Many business organizations dealing with healthcare face additional ethical issues because of the sensitivity in the matter (Wallace 15). Such importance is part of the reason why the formation of a Compliance Department is crucial especially when research is being undertaken. However, for any compliance and oversight practice to be effective in its mandate and operations, it must be fitted into the main entity's organizational structure. The process and results of such a consideration are as important as the compliance department's mandate.

Most large considerations assume the common organizational structure that includes a Chief Operations Officer (COO). This executive is responsible for the coordination of all the firm's operational departments and their coordinative efforts in achieving the organization's objective. Consequently, the formation of a Research Compliance Department for the organization this paper targets would obviously involve the identification and recruitment of a Chief Compliance Officer (CCO). This executive would be in charge of the entire Research Compliance Department and its operations in a manner that the Chief Executive Officer (CEO) is to the entire organizations. However, with regard to whom the Compliance Department answers to in the main organization or organizational structure, the CCO would be answerable to the COO, who is in turn answerable to the CEO.

Some business organizations are not as large meaning that they do not include a Chief Operations Officer (COO). Such business organizations have executives that manage entire departments as Managing Directors and sit at Boards of Directors. Some examples of these executives include the Chief Finance Officer (CFO), Chief Technical Officer (CTO), and the Chief Marketing Officer (CMO). All these executives are directly answerable to the CEO. Applying this rationale to the main organization the intended Research Compliance Department intends to serve, one discovers that the Chief Compliance Officer who will head this new department must be directly answerable to the CEO.

Other business organizations might decide to create entirely new department to serve new interests brought about by expansion, mergers or even research. In such circumstances, the team tasked with identifying and recruiting the heads of these departments must also create unique spaces according to the roles the new departments will serve in the main organization. Therefore, a newly created Research Compliance Department would be stationed in the main organization's head quarters where the department would operate from a C-suite. Applying this rationale to the main organization the paper focuses on, one find that the Research Compliance Department would be stationed at the firm's headquarters in the wing aptly named the C-suite. This department's head would be a Chief Compliance Officer (CCO), whose mandate as head of a completely independent department would be to manage the oversight and compliance issues related to the main organization's research activities.

THE PRIMARY ETHICAL CONCERNS AFFECTING THE PROCESS

During the formation of the Research Compliance Department intended to provide additional oversight to the organization intent on healthcare research, the executives must carefully consider certain ethical concerns pertinent to the process. The first ethical concern that the Chief Compliance Officer and his team must consider is the entry of bad management into the research ranks (Wallace 53). Research activity, especially those targeting the healthcare industry, is a critical process that demands personnel with the highest integrity. Therefore, the CCO must make appropriate action to prevent the entry of researchers that have demonstrated unethical behavior in the past. Some characteristics the CCO might need to check out for among the team involved in the research endeavor include dishonesty, recklessness, and disrespect.

The second ethical concern that the Research Compliance Department's head might need to consider revolves around training and education (Tsan and Tsan 224). Most large companies that declare an intention to carry out research attract a large pool of professionals drawn by the opportunities for growth, innovation, and attractive remunerations. Many cases have come up in the past where some of these prospective employees have cheated the Human Resources and Compliance Departments about their training and education in order to gain entry into these attractive opportunities.

Another ethical concern that the CCO must check during his tenure as head of the organization's Research Compliance Department is unfair performance incentives and rewards. Some organizations attempt to inspire their research personnel using unfair or even untenable performance incentives and rewards that may include bribes and promises. Such practices constitute unethical behavior given the sensitivity of the industry the research endeavor targets. Research activity and process in the healthcare sectors must be allowed its fair share of time in order to ensure that no corners are cut or mistakes missed (Wallace 15). Therefore, the CCO must watch out for unethical issues related to unfair performance incentives and rewards to prevent compromising both the process and results of the research process.

All research endeavors that aim to introduce new innovations or make significant improvement in the healthcare industry rely on a solid financial backing. However, the creation of a large pool of resources for processes of innovation introduces ethical issues related to financial integrity because researchers can get away with unforeseen costs. Therefore, the head of the Research Compliance Department must liaise with the Financial Department to ensure that auditing and financial oversight is done well. Many research processes or initiatives in the past have suffered large financial losses and compromised ethical standing due to reckless auditing. Therefore, as head of research compliance, the CCO must be keen to ensure no ethical issued related to finances arise.

No compliance and oversight practice is complete until it creates, communicates and implements solid disciplinary measures for all wrong doers as part of its ethical sustainability strategy. The organization that is keen to engage in research and tasks a Research Compliance Department with the job must also include some strategy to ensure that all disciplinary issues are tackled accordingly. Mishandling such issues introduces serious ethical concerns in the process where large pools or resources and strict objectives are involved. Therefore, the CCO must identify, communicate, and implement a strict disciplinary regime to prevent such ethical concerns from becoming reality.

HOW THE COMPLIANCE DEPARTMENT WOULD MAINTAIN OVERSIGHT OF RESEARCH OPERATIONS

Unlike most business operations, innovation and research present the management of business organizations with challenges in the form of difficulties in predictions touching on time, impact, and steps necessary. However, the definitions of research compliance revolve around one central theme; the guidance of research activity and decisions in using organizational resources to deliver value through innovation, to meet preset organization goals, and build optimized competitive advantages in the competitive health or technology industries or markets (Tsan and Tsan 225). Ideally, the main goal according to this school of thought is management decisions that improve research performance.

In the course of trying to maintain oversight over the research operations, the Research Compliance Department would strive to direct its vast pool of resources to create more layers of oversight in order to add value for its organization, create more competitive advantage and better achieve its organizational goals. In order for the Compliance Department's management has succeed in the process, a compliance strategy is necessary. It is a continuous process that needs constant input from all players. Within the realms of research, the physicians and researchers are always shifting their needs meaning that resources and other similar needs need to be aligned with these changes (Wallace 53). However, these needs need to be observed and audited carefully to ensure that the process does not deplete its allocated resources pool in a reckless manner.

Many compliance managers consider manpower as a potentially strategic tool in maintaining oversight in research processes, some scholars have gone a step further to suggest the existence of similar strategic abilities in executing oversight over the personnel involved. Some researchers have argued that many organizations acquire distinct and measurable quantity indicators in their research endeavors based on their knowledge of how to strategically man the process (Tsan and Tsan 225). Most organizations simply man their research processes with little regard for oversight and instead concentrate on experience, training and the outcome. However, oversight of the process depends on maintaining a small but effective team that can easily and cost effectively be observed for the sake of maintaining oversight over the entire research process. Therefore, the main healthcare-oriented organization could benefit from its Compliance Department's head liaising with the HRM team to maintain a lean team in the research department to optimize oversight.

Quality Indicators prove the Compliance Department of any major organization involved in research with tools to maintain oversight in their processes. These indicators identify and mark portions of certain organizational processes, strategies, or even products that have demonstrated high quality thus creating some degree of accountability (Wallace 15). The healthcare organization involved in research could create and maintain a good degree of oversight in their processes by inducting certain quality markets aligned with the organization's predetermined objectives. Therefore, the CCO would identify these markers as they come up and mark them as indicators of accountability thus maintaining oversight in the entire research process.

TOOLS AND APPROACHES USABLE IN THE ORGANIZATION AND THEIR EFFECTIVENESS

One approach towards the creation and implementation is the use of a standards and sustainability strategy. This strategy offers the firm a higher competitive advantage in terms of the characteristics of its end-product relative to the research process and product. Arguably, the firm may be engaged in healthcare goods or services that resemble those of its rivals, but how it executes its innovation process is influenced a lot by the Compliance Department's strategies. Research demonstrates that even the most subtle changes in the oversight process that firms make in competitive markets can make the difference. Therefore, these changes, and how they are optimized to offer customers the most value constitute such strategies for competitive advantage.

Many jurisdictions offer a set of guidelines that healthcare organizations intent on carrying out research must follow to implement compliance and oversight over these processes. One such organization that offers tools and advice to these organizations in the United States is the Human Research Protection Program (HRPP) (Tsan and Tsan 225). This organization not only monitors all human research endeavors, but also offers implementation advice and tools to organizations intent on such endeavors. Therefore, the parent organization in conjunction with its Research Compliance Department's CCO could use these tools and approaches as both a method of adhering with best industry practices and effective implementation.

The organization could also use process-based plans and action plans to not only introduce effectiveness in the research compliance practice, but also the research process itself. Such considerations not only contribute to distinct competitive advantage in innovation but also include processes and plans that marry into a workable strategic change. Although the healthcare organization may face little threat in the way of rivalry in its large scale healthcare sector, other areas of its core business have continued to be slowly consumed by newer and smaller but intensely innovative companies. However, the company can tap into some of its core strengths such as economies of scale and better technical experience to ensure that although the products and markets are similar, the execution is better. Such action plans also complement its research compliance and oversight practice very well.

The management team chosen also offers the research compliance and oversight program with another tool that they could use to maintain effective oversight of the entire process. Choosing experienced and well trained CCOs, and other pertinent personnel also contributes to the oversight process by delivering capable manpower into the process or compliance and oversight management. Such tools also constitute a strategic approach for competitive advantage in research where unique intellectual property is created and optimized for both human benefit and commercial applications. Because of such knowledgeable CCO's , the company is not only able to carry out research effectively, but also offer the customers better goods and services, it also acquires the ability to surpass its rivals and perform relatively better.

The creation of a quality control and assurance mandate, or subscription to an international quality assurance measurement also offers the Research Compliance Department with another approach to optimizing its operations (Wallace 16). Most schools of thought and research endeavors into the most appropriate business practices in terms of research support quality assurance strategies as approaches to succeeding in terms of compliance and oversight. These schools of thought agree that the longevity of businesses is almost as important as the sustenance of profitability and operations. However, in order to initiate sustainable strategy, various considerations must be made for the sake of success within the context of customer welfare.

If the parent organization is a multinational, its compliance practice would benefit immensely from engaging in the main organization's sustainable strategy. Such moves benefit the compliance department in many ways that includes investing in scientific education institutions that are the main source of its skills (Wallace 53). It also invests in environmental programs worldwide given the need for both CSR and environmental conservation. Such activities provide the Compliance Department with an edge socially thus demonstrating their dedication in-house and around the organization as well. Although these approaches are part of the multinational's extensive sustainability strategy aimed at not only creating value for its stakeholders, but demonstrating willingness for future growth that is both considerate and strategic, they offer its research compliance department a great optimization tool.

The CCO could also argue that sustainable value is sustainable strategy based on his 2X2 model's ability to introduce efficiency to the business environment. By pitting internal factors at both the parent company and his Compliance Department against external ones, and the present against the future the CCO may succeed in demonstrating the manner in which the right mix serves the present state of affairs while contemplating about the future for both the stakeholders and shareholders. This interesting school of thought has clear indications of an efficiency strategy although some scholars argued that sustainability cannot be function of such few variables (Tsan and Tsan 227). In deed the 2X2 model could offer the Research Compliance Department with some marginal uses, but the actual applicability must be the CCO's management decision based on the actual research endeavor. However, a clear understanding of the applicability of these theoretical schools of thought and adept managerial strategy will shore the company into a successful future.

HOW TO INDUCT THE PERSONNEL INVOLVED INTO THE NOTION OF ADDITIONAL LAYERS OF OVERSIGHT

Both the parent organization and the Research Compliance Department must identify methods of convincing the personnel involved in the research processes to accept the additional layers of oversight. One of the most common and effective methods usable in this context is the communication of a culture of accountability. Because the healthcare organization must have invested vast resources into the research process, the CCO might want to encourage his department to communicate the need for accountability to the researchers and physicians involved in the parent organization's research endeavor. Such strategy would form the first action towards the Compliance Department's intentions of convincing the personnel to accept the additional layers of oversight.

Many organizations implement their oversight practices using invasive technological approaches such as large CCTV systems and ambiguous security checks. Such strategies could work in high risk environments such as the banking or intelligence research sectors. However, in order to convince researchers and physicians involved in healthcare research to accept additional layers of research, more subtle approaches might be necessary. One approach that could work would be the abandonment of invasive monitoring technology such as visible CCTV systems with biometric access systems. Physicians and other researchers would accept the additional layers of oversight better if all they needed were palm-prints and eye scans to access restricted areas of the research area compared to black ugly CCTV systems monitoring their every move. Therefore, the CCO might be well advised to adopt less invasive monitoring systems as a way of convincing the research personnel involved to accept the additional layers of oversight.

Many compliance managers consider manpower as a potentially strategic tool in maintaining oversight in research processes although some scholars have gone a step further to suggest the existence of similar strategic abilities in executing oversight over smaller numbers of personnel. Some researchers have argued that many organizations acquire distinct and measurable acceptance advantages in their Research Compliance Departments based on strategically manning the processes. Most organizations simply man their research processes with little regard for oversight and instead concentrate on experience, training and the outcome. However, oversight of the process depends on maintaining a small but effective team that can easily and cost effectively be observed for the sake of maintaining oversight over the entire research process (Wallace 16). Therefore, the main healthcare-oriented organization could benefit from its Compliance Department's head liaising with the HRM team to maintain a lean team in the research department to optimize oversight.

Incentives and reward systems provide the management of organizations with an effective method of managing human resources and controlling their actions. A similar rationale could be used to convince the personnel involved in the research processes of a healthcare organization where there is a Research Compliance Department. The Department's CCO may initiate such acceptance by communicating certain rewards available only to personnel under his department's oversight who not only accept the practice, but follow it well. If implemented well, such a strategy would not only enroll more research personnel into the additional layers of oversight, but also convince them to adhere to the compliance processes and requirements.

Another effective method of convincing personnel in any professional setting to accept additional requirements such as additional layers of oversight is to induct such requirements in training requirements. By making recommendations that include Compliance training and oversight management in on-the-job training regimens, the organizations convinces the personnel to accept these layers thus circumventing the problems associated with human resources and oversight (Wallace 16). The parent company and its Research Compliance Department's CCO could make the requirement for compliance training mandatory for all prospective personnel interested in the research process. Such maneuvers would succeed in convincing the personnel to embrace additional oversight as part of the requirements package.

CONCLUSION

When the management of a healthcare organization tasks the VC of healthcare systems with forming a research compliance department, there are many consideration the executive must make in order to be effective in that capacity. As part of the large organization involved in among other activities healthcare, various ethical issues arise that necessitate the creation of such a department. However, the process is not easy as many considerations have to be made.

This paper analyzed the process of creating a Research Compliance Program by investigating the process of creating a Research Compliance Department using a distinct set of considerations. These considerations include who the compliance department answers to, the primary ethical issues involved, how the department intends to maintain oversight, the tools and approaches applicable as well as their applicability, and to assimilate all personnel involved into the notion of additional oversight.

Works Cited

Tsan, Min-Fu, and Linda W. Tsan. "Assessing the quality of human research protection programs to improve protection of human subjects participating in clinical trials." *Clinical Trials*, vol. 12, no. 3, 2015, pp. 224-231.

Wallace, Marsha C. "Practical Considerations and Approaches to Developing an Internal Compliance Auditing and Monitoring Program for Human Subject Research." *Journal of Health Care Compliance*, Dec. 2015, pp. 15-54, *Aspen Publishers Inc.*. Accessed 5 May 2017.